AF442878

Contents

What Is the Liver?

The liver is the largest solid organ in the body. People may not know that the liver is also the largest gland in the body. The liver is actually two different types of gland. It is a secretory gland because it has a specialized structure that is designed to allow it to make and secrete bile into the bile ducts. It also is an endocrine gland since it makes and secretes chemicals directly into the blood that have effects on other organs in the body. Bile is a fluid that both aids in digestion and absorption of fats as well as carries waste products into the intestine.

Where Is Liver Located?

The liver is located just below the diaphragm (the muscular membrane separating the chest from the abdomen), primarily in the upper right part of the abdomen, mostly under the ribs. However, it also extends across the middle of the upper abdomen and part way into the left upper abdomen. An irregularly shaped, dome-like solid structure, the liver consists of two main parts (a larger right lobe and a smaller left lobe) and two minor lobes. As you can see in the diagram below, the upper border of the right lobe is at the level of the top of the 5th rib (a little less than 1/2 inch below the nipple), and the upper border of the left lobe is just below the 5th rib (about 3/4 inch below the nipple). During inspiration (breathing in), the liver is pushed down by the diaphragm and the lower edge of the liver descends below the margin of the lowest rib (costal margin).

How Big Is the Liver?

The liver weighs about three and a half pounds (1.6 kilograms). It measures on average, about 8 inches (20 cm) horizontally (across), and 6.5 inches (17 cm) vertically (down), and is 4.5 inches (12 cm) thick.

What Does the Liver Do?

The liver has a multitude of important and complex functions. Some of these functions are to:

- Manufacture (synthesize) proteins, including albumin (to help maintain the volume of blood) and blood clotting factors

- Synthesize, store, and process (metabolize) fats, including fatty acids (used for energy) and cholesterol

- Metabolize and store carbohydrates, which are used as the source for the sugar (glucose) in blood that red blood cells and the brain use
- Form and secrete bile that contains bile acids to aid in the intestinal absorption of fats and the fat-soluble vitamins A, D, E, and K.
- Eliminate, by metabolizing and/or secreting, the potentially harmful biochemical products produced by the body, such as bilirubin from the breakdown of old red blood cells, and ammonia from the breakdown of proteins
- Detoxify, by metabolizing and/or secreting, drugs, alcohol, and environmental toxins

What Are the Special Features of the Liver?

The liver has many special features. For example, in order to carry out its secretory functions, ducts (tubes) closely connect it to the gallbladder and intestines. Thus, bile made by the liver travels through these tubes to the gallbladder. The bile is stored in the gallbladder between meals, and then is discharged into the intestines at mealtime to aid in digestion.

For another example, the liver is appropriately situated in the body to directly receive the blood that comes from the intestines (portal blood). With this arrangement, the liver can readily process (metabolize) nutrients absorbed from food as well as other contents of the portal blood. Indeed, because of its numerous biochemical functions, the liver is considered the biochemical factory of the body.

Further, the liver is organized strategically to coordinate its structure, including its blood circulation, with its functions. Four key features of this organization of the liver are as follows.

1. The basic unit of the liver is called an acinus (pronounced as "i-nus: plural acini", there are numerous acini in the liver.) In each acinus, the liver cells (hepatocytes) are grouped into three zones that are anatomically related to the liver's blood supply and drainage. Thus, the blood enters zone one first, and then travels through the second and third zones before leaving the liver. Each zone has its own special functions to

perform. (Moreover, because of these different functions, as well as the different relationships to the flow of blood, the zones have different susceptibilities to injury.)

2. Specialized areas of the walls of adjacent liver cells (hepatocytes) join to form bile canaliculi (pronounced kan" ah-lik' u-li). The canaliculi are microscopic tubes that transport bile that is produced by the liver cells (hepatocytes). Then, meeting with other canaliculi, they ultimately empty into tiny bile ducts. These bile ducts join with other bile ducts to form larger bile ducts that ultimately leave the liver.

3. The liver has a unique, dual blood supply. One comes from the portal vein, as already mentioned, and the other from the hepatic

artery. The hepatic artery brings to the liver oxygenated blood that comes from the lungs, heart, and branches of the aorta. So, finally, tiny branches of the portal vein and hepatic artery travel in the liver together with the tiny bile ducts in tracts called portal tracts (triads).

4. The hepatic artery supplies blood to nourish the bile ducts and the liver cells (hepatocytes). This blood joins with the portal vein blood in tiny blood vessels called sinusoids. The sinusoids are situated on each side of single-cell-thick plates of liver cells (hepatocytes), and they have an exceptionally porous lining. This unique arrangement enables passage of even large molecules (for example, lipoproteins) through the sinusoidal lining to and from the liver cells (hepatocytes). The blood travels in the sinusoids

through the three acinar zones. Finally, the blood is drained from the liver by the hepatic veins and then heads back to the heart and lungs.

What Are the Early Signs and Symptoms of Liver Disease?

Acute and chronic liver diseases can interfere with the functions of the liver and thereby cause symptoms. However, the liver has a hefty reserve capacity. In other words, it usually takes substantial damage to the liver before a disease interferes with the functions of the liver and causes symptoms. Examples of such symptoms are:

- Jaundice (yellow skin) that can occur when the liver is unable to properly metabolize or secrete the yellow pigment bilirubin in bile
- Bleeding or easy bruising that can occur when the liver is unable to make enough of the normal blood clotting proteins
- Swelling of the legs with fluid (edema) that can occur when the liver is unable to make enough albumin and the serum albumin gets too low
- Fatigue that is of unknown cause, but may be related to some impaired metabolic function of the liver

What Are the Common Types of Liver Disease?

The most common liver diseases are various types of:

1. acute (sudden) hepatitis (inflammation),

2. chronic (long duration) hepatitis,

3. fatty liver disease,

4. cirrhosis (scarring), and

5. cancer.

Cancers that affect the liver are most commonly metastatic cancers that have spread via the bloodstream to the liver from other sites in the body. However, primary cancers (cancers that arise in the liver) can also occur. The most common type of primary liver cancers are known as hepatocellular carcinomas.

Common causes of liver disease include:

1. viruses,

2. drugs - prescription, over-the-counter (OTC), herbal supplements, vitamins, and dietary supplements (for example, acetaminophen [Tylenol and others],

3. alcohol,

4. metabolic problems,

5. immune (defense) system, and

6. genetic (hereditary) abnormalities.

But note that, contrary to a popular misconception, alcohol is only one of the many causes of liver disease. Moreover, sometimes the cause of the liver disease is not known.

What can help with improving your liver health?

Your everyday choices and lifestyle habits can affect the health of your liver in the long term. While these strategies may not seem as simple as a one-time cleanse, they're more likely to protect your liver and keep it healthy.

Let's look at seven key strategies that can help protect your liver in your daily life.

1. Limit your alcohol consumption

Your liver processes every alcoholic beverage you consume, including wine, beer, and spirits.

The more you drink, the harder your liver has to work.

Over time, excessive drinking can take a toll, destroying liver cells. Alcohol-related liver disease (ARLD) includes several liver different conditions, such as:

- alcoholic fatty liver disease
- acute alcoholic hepatitis
- alcoholic cirrhosis

To avoid alcohol-related liver disease, follow the recommendations for alcohol outlined in the 2015–2020 Dietary Guidelines for AmericansTrusted Source. That's one drink per day for women and two drinks per day for men.

A standard drink is considered to be:

- 12 fluid ounces (fl. oz.) of regular beer (about 5 percent alcohol)
- 8 to 9 fl. oz. of malt liquor (about 7 percent alcohol)
- 5 fl. oz. of wine (about 12 percent alcohol)
- 1.5 fl. oz. shot of distilled spirits like gin, rum, tequila, whiskey (about 40 percent alcohol)

In addition, avoid mixing alcohol and medication, which puts excess strain on your liver.

2. Monitor your use of medications

All medications — whether they're over the counter or prescribed by a doctor — eventually pass through your liver where they're broken down.

Most medications are safe for your liver when taken as directed. However, taking too much of a drug, taking it too often, taking the wrong type, or taking several drugs at once can harm your liver.

Acetaminophen (Tylenol) is an example of a common over-the-counter medication that can have serious consequences for your liver when taken incorrectly.

You should never take more than 1,000 milligrams (mg) of acetaminophen at a time, or exceed the maximum dose of 3,000 mg per day. Don't mix acetaminophen and alcohol.

If you're concerned about how a medication may affect your liver, talk to your doctor or pharmacist. You can also ask to have your liver tested before and after starting a new medication.

3. Don't assume supplements are good for your liver

Like medications, supplements such as vitamins, minerals, herbs, and natural remedies are processed by your liver.

Just because a product is natural doesn't mean it won't have long-term consequences for your liver. In fact, many seemingly harmless products are capable of doing damage.

A 2017 article published in the journal Gastroenterology & HepatologyTrusted Source identifies performance-enhancing and weight loss supplements as potentially harmful to the liver. Green tea extract is another common herbal supplement that may affect your liver.

Even vitamins, in particular vitamin A and niacin, can cause liver damage if you take too much of them.

To avoid liver complications, talk to your doctor before taking supplements.

4. Adopt a liver-friendly diet

This shouldn't come as a surprise, but your diet plays a significant role in the overall health of your liver.

To ensure your diet is benefiting your liver in the long term, try the following:

- Eat a variety of foods. Choose whole grains, fruits and vegetables, lean protein, dairy, and healthy fats. Foods such as grapefruit, blueberries, nuts, and fatty fish are known to have potential benefits for the liver.

- Get enough fiber. Fiber is essential to helping your liver function smoothly. Fruits and vegetables and whole grains are great sources of fiber to incorporate into your diet.

- Stay hydrated. Make sure you drink enough water each day to keep your liver in tip-top shape.

- Limit fatty, sugary, and salty foods. Foods that are high in fat, sugar, and salt can affect liver function over time. Fried and fast foods can also affect the health of your liver.

- Drink coffee. Coffee has been shownTrusted Source to lower the risk of liver diseases such as cirrhosis and liver cancer. It works by preventing the accumulation of fat and collagen, two factors in liver disease.

5. Exercise regularly

Physical activity isn't just good for your musculoskeletal and cardiovascular systems. It's also good for your liver.

Research from 2018Trusted Source examined the role of exercise in non-alcoholic fatty liver disease (NAFLD), now one of the most common liver diseases.

The researchers concluded that both cardio and resistance exercises help to prevent fat buildup in the liver. Fat buildup is associated with NAFLD.

You don't need to run marathons to reap the benefits. You can start exercising today by taking a brisk walk, doing an online workout class, or going on a bike ride.

6. Take precautions against hepatitis

Hepatitis is a disease that causes liver inflammation. Some types of hepatitis only cause acute, short-term symptoms (hepatitis A), while others are long-term illnesses (hepatitis B and C).

You can protect yourself against hepatitis by first understanding how the most common forms spread.

- Hepatitis A is transmitted by consuming food or water contaminated with the feces of someone who has hepatitis A.

- Hepatitis B is transmitted through contact with bodily fluids from someone who has hepatitis B. Bodily fluids include blood, vaginal discharge, and semen.

- Hepatitis C is transmitted through contact with bodily fluids from someone who has hepatitis C.

To protect yourself against hepatitis, you can:

- Practice good hygiene. Wash your hands regularly and use hand sanitizer.

- Take extra precautions when traveling. Learn more about hepatitis risks in the region you're visiting. Avoid local tap water or ice and unwashed fruit or vegetables.

- Don't share personal items. Keep your toothbrush and razor to yourself. If you use intravenous (IV) drugs, don't share needles.

- Make sure needles are sterilized. Before getting a tattoo or piercing, make sure the studio uses disposable needles or an autoclave machine to sterilize needles.

• Practice safer sex. If you have sex with more than one partner, use a condom to lower your risk of hepatitis B and C.

• Get vaccinated. Vaccination can help you avoid contracting hepatitis A and B. There's currently no vaccine for hepatitis C.

7. Limit your contact with environmental toxins

Not only does your liver process chemicals that enter your body through your mouth, but it also processes chemicals that enter through your nose and skin.

Some everyday household products contain toxins that can damage your liver, especially if you come into contact with them regularly.

To prevent long-term damage to your liver, opt for organic cleaning products and techniques to clean your home. Avoid using pesticides and herbicides in your yard, or take precautions to avoid inhaling chemical fumes.

If you must use chemicals or aerosols inside the house — to paint, for instance — make sure your space is well ventilated. If that's not possible, wear a mask.

Top foods and drinks for liver health

Some of the best foods and drinks that are good for the liver include:

1. Coffee

A 2013 review that appears in the journal Liver International suggests that over 50 percent of people in the United States consume coffee daily.

Coffee appears to be good for the liver, especially because it protects against issues such as fatty liver disease.

The review also notes that daily coffee intake may help reduce the risk of chronic liver disease. It may also protect the liver from damaging conditions, such as liver cancer.

A 2014 study that appears in the Journal of Clinical Gastroenterology suggests that the protective effects of coffee are due to how it influences liver enzymes.

Coffee, it reports, seems to reduce fat buildup in the liver. It also increases protective antioxidants in the liver. Compounds in coffee also help liver enzymes rid the body of cancer-causing substances.

2. Oatmeal

Consuming oatmeal is an easy way to add fiber to the diet. Fiber is an important tool for digestion, and the specific fibers in oats may be especially helpful for the liver. Oats and oatmeal are high in compounds called beta-glucans.

As a 2017 study in the International Journal of Molecular Sciences reports, beta-glucans are very biologically active in the body. They help modulate the immune system and fight against inflammation, and they may be especially helpful in the fight against diabetes and obesity.

The review also notes that beta-glucans from oats appear to help reduce the amount of fat stored in the liver in mice, which could also help protect the liver. More clinical studies are necessary to confirm this, however.

People looking to add oats or oatmeal to their diet should look for whole oats or steel-cut oats, rather than prepackaged oatmeal. Prepackaged oatmeal may contain fillers such as flour or sugars, which will not be as beneficial for the body.

3. Green tea

A 2016 review in the journal Nutrition suggests that green tea may help reduce the risk of liver cancer in female Asian populations.

It is important to note that tea may be better than extracts, as some extracts may damage the liver rather than heal it.

However, the study notes that more research is necessary.

4. Garlic

Adding garlic to the diet may also help stimulate the liver. A 2016 study that appears in the journal Advanced Biomedical Research notes that garlic consumption reduces body weight and fat content in people with NAFLD, with no changes to lean body mass. This is beneficial, as being overweight or obese is a contributing factor to NAFLD.

5. Berries

Many dark berries, such as blueberries, raspberries, and cranberries, contain antioxidants called polyphenols, which may help protect the liver from damage.

As a study in the World Journal of Gastroenterology suggests, regularly eating berries may also help stimulate the immune system.

6. Grapes

The study that features in the World Journal of Gastroenterology reports that grapes, grape juice, and grape seeds are rich in antioxidants that may help the liver by reducing inflammation and preventing liver damage.

Eating whole, seeded grapes is a simple way to add these compounds to the diet. A grape seed extract supplement may also provide antioxidants.

7. Grapefruit

The World Journal of Gastroenterology study also mentions grapefruit as a helpful food. Grapefruit contains two primary antioxidants: naringin and naringenin. These may help protect the liver from injury by reducing inflammation and protecting the liver cells.

The compounds may also reduce fat buildup in the liver and increase the enzymes that burn fat. This may make grapefruit a helpful tool in the fight against NAFLD.

8. Prickly pear

The fruit and juice of the prickly pear may also be beneficial to liver health. The World Journal of Gastroenterology study suggests that compounds in the fruit may help protect the organ.

Most research focuses on extracts from the fruit, however, so studies that focus on the fruit or juice itself are necessary.

9. Plant foods in general

A 2015 study that appears in the journal Evidence-based Complementary and Alternative Medicine reports that a large number of plant foods may be helpful for the liver.

These include:

- avocado
- banana
- barley
- beets and beet juice
- broccoli
- brown rice

- carrots
- fig
- greens such as kale and collards
- lemon
- papaya
- watermelon

People should eat these foods as part of a whole and balanced diet.

10. Fatty fish

As a study in the World Journal of Gastroenterology points out, consuming fatty fish and fish oil supplements may help reduce the impact of conditions such as NAFLD.

Fatty fish is rich in omega-3 fatty acids, which are the good fats that help reduce inflammation.

These fats may be especially helpful in the liver, as they appear to prevent the buildup of excess fats and maintain enzyme levels in the liver.

The study recommends eating oily fish two or more times each week. If it is not easy to incorporate fatty fish such as herring or salmon into the diet, try taking a daily fish oil supplement.

11. Nuts

The same study says that eating nuts may be another simple way to keep the liver healthy and protect against NAFLD. Nuts generally contain unsaturated fatty acids, vitamin E, and antioxidants. These compounds may help prevent NAFLD, as well as reduce inflammation and oxidative stress.

Eating a handful of nuts, such as walnuts or almonds, each day may help maintain liver health. People should be sure not to eat too many, however, as nuts are high in calories.

12. Olive oil

Eating too much fat is not good for the liver, but some fats may help it. According to the World Journal of Gastroenterology study, adding olive oil to the diet may help reduce oxidative stress and improve liver function. This is due to the high content of unsaturated fatty acids in the oil.

Foods to avoid

In general, finding balance in the diet will keep the liver healthy. However, there are also some foods and food groups that the liver finds harder to process. These include:

- Fatty foods: These include fried foods, fast food, and takeout from many restaurants. Packaged snacks, chips, and nuts may also be surprisingly high in fats.

- Starchy foods: These include breads, pasta, and cakes or baked goods.

- Sugar: Cutting back on sugar and sugary foods such as cereals, baked goods, and candies may help reduce the stress on the liver.

- Salt: Simple ways to reduce salt intake include eating out less, avoiding canned meats or vegetables, and reducing or avoiding salted deli meats and bacon.

- Alcohol: Anyone looking to give their liver a break should consider reducing their intake of alcohol or eliminating it from the diet completely.

Liver Rescue Diet

Liver Rescue is a 9-day protocol of healthy meals that are supposed to super-boost the liver. Medical Medium explains that the liver is responsible for over 2,000 chemical functions in the body. The liver is incredibly smart and knows how to clear out the bad and take in the good. He also explains that in our modern life, the liver can get overburdened. This can be due to chemicals, foods we eat, alcohol, tobacco, nicotine, etc. When this happens, we may start to experience symptoms like unexpected weight gain, bloating, trouble digesting, IBS, acne, depression, anxiety and so on. Therefore, cleansing the liver can help it restore some of its strength and help the body function as normal again.

The Liver Rescue is also considered an emotional detox. Medical Medium explains that the liver also stores a lot of unprocessed emotions in the liver. When you cleanse in this way, a lot of emotions will rise to the surface. You might also experience a lot of fatigue and tiredness as a part of the cleanse, in addition to anger, restlessness and some weird dreams (talking from experience).

Why Liver Rescue?

One of the reasons we wanted to do this cleanse was that individually we were experiencing some health issues such as digestive issues, anxiety and hormonal imbalances causing bacterial acne and a disappearing cycle. These have been reoccurring health issues that have gotten better over the years, but that we haven't quite gotten to the bottom of. That's why cleanses are so good, because they give you a chance to start over. And this one is actually more of a meal plan than a cleanse.

How does the Liver Rescue Diet work?

The Liver Rescue diet is divided into three parts. The intention behind this is to slowly ease into the cleanse and then out again without stressing the liver.

The 3 - Easing in

The first three days you are supposed to eat quite similar to what you would normally do, except that you should avoid gluten, dairy, eggs, lamb, pork products and canola oil. You are also supposed to reduce your consumption of radical fats (nuts, seeds, oils, coconut, animal protein, etc.) by 50 %, and wait to eat fats until dinner. If you eat animal products, these should be eaten at dinner, and only one serving. Your focus should be bringing in more and more fruits, veggies and leafy greens each day!

The 6 - Time to clean

The next three days the real cleansing begins. These days you follow a more strict protocol on what to eat, and you do not eat any fat these days (including healthy fats like avocado, nuts, seeds, coconut oil). You also eat a LOT of food and you are not supposed to be hungry!

The salads portions are pretty big, and you are supposed to eat a lot of apples during the day. These were also the hardest days of the cleanse.

The 9 - Time to shine

The last three days are supposed to be the time when the toxins are ready to be flushed out! These days the food was finally mixed up a bit, and instead of having the same salad for lunch, we had a really delicious spinach soup with cucumber noodles. After the first day of the 9, we both felt a huge relief and really felt that this detox was working. It was still hard to digest everything, so we did yin yoga every night, and made sure to do lots of breathing exercises. It was also very motivating knowing we were almost done. For dinner day 7, you even get steamed potatoes, which was so nice and comforting.

The last day - day 9 was the day you flush it all out. You drink liquids all day and try to take it easy.

The 7-Day Detox Diet Plan: Time to Get Healthy & Active

Detox Diet Plan: Five days before you begin your detox diet plan, progressively eliminate alcohol, coffee, cigarettes, refined sugars, saturated fats and all processed foods.

Smooth digestion and absorption of nutrients along with your liver's efficient processing of toxins are absolutely critical for great health. That's why a cleanse program can be a powerful tool to rejuvenate your body and skin from the inside out. The key to comfortable cleanse is to ease yourself into the program, so that your body doesn't go into a shock. Five days before you begin your detox diet plan, progressively eliminate alcohol, coffee, cigarettes, refined sugars, saturated fats and all processed foods. These can add as toxins in your body, and must be removed from the diet at all costs.

Increase fiber intake to help keep your colon clean. Along with the fiber from fruits and vegetables, include two tablespoon of chia seeds in a glass of water to eliminate toxins from your body. Don't forget to drink lots of filtered water- at least eight glasses per day. This will further help the process of detoxification in your body.

DAY 1

Start the morning with half a lemon squeezed into warm water or cleansing herb tea. Follow with a brisk walk, bike ride, yoga or swimming.

BREAKFAST: Fresh vegetables juice (choose from the list below)

- Carrots
- Beetroot
- Celery
- Mint
- Coriander
- Parsley
- Wheatgrass
- Spinach
- Kale
-

Add a tablespoon of chia seeds to your juice, for that extra fiber and power boost. (I don't recommend juicing fruits as that will shoot up your sugar levels and we don't want that happening).

LUNCH: Raw or lightly steamed vegetables with a variety of seasonal preferably organic vegetables .You can choose from the following:

- Mushrooms
- Spinach
- Mustard leaves
- Fenugreek leaves
- Beetroot

- Broccoli
- Cabbage
- Capsicums
- Pumpkins
- Carrots
- Onions
- Garlic
- Ginger

DINNER: Vegetable stew

In a large saucepan, saute onions and garlic. Then add your favourite veggies, saute for another 2 minutes. Add 2 cups of filtered water and sea salt. Slow cook till the veggies are done. You could blend the ingredients for a thick broth or eat it as is with chunks of veggies.

SNACKS: Drink as much water, unsweetened herbal tea as you wish during the day. Aim for at least 8 glass of water within the day. Make a trail mix of nuts and seeds like walnuts, almonds, pumpkin seeds, sunflower seeds, melon seeds, chia seeds and flax seeds. Eat low GI fruits like guava, pear, apple, orange, strawberries, peach, plums and apricots.

DAY 2

Start the morning with half a lemon squeezed into warm water or cleansing herb tea. Follow with a brisk walk, bike ride, yoga or swimming

BREAKFAST: Fresh vegetable juice with 1 table spoon of chia seeds blended in. Choose from the list of juicing vegetables provided earlier.

LUNCH: Lightly cooked vegetables with quinoa and baby spinach salad.

DINNER: Vegetable stew with stir-fried red and yellow capsicums and broccoli, tossed with extra virgin olive oil, lemon juice and garlic.

ANY TIME SNACKS: Choose from the snack list given for Day 1.

DAY 3

Start the morning with half a lemon squeezed into warm water or cleansing herb tea. Follow with a brisk walk, bike ride, yoga or swimming.

BREAKFAST: 3/4 of cup of natural yoghurt with sliced fresh fruits, sprinkle with chia seeds, sliced almonds and walnuts and drizzle with a little raw honey if desired. You can follow this with green tea or herb tea.

LUNCH: Lentil and Vegetable Stew

Saute 1/2 cup of yellow moong dal, 1 cup of your favourite veggies, small pieces of ginger and two cloves of garlic in some extra virgin olive oil. Add 2 cups of water and salt to taste. Slow cook till the dal and veggies are done, garnish with coriander or parsley.

DINNER: Raw Papaya and Carrot Salad

Toss 2 cups of lettuce, 1 grated carrot and 1/2 raw papaya together. Mix 1 tablespoon of balsamic vinegar and 1 tablespoon of extra virgin olive oil, fresh lemon juice and drizzle over the top.

ANY TIME SNACKS: Choose from the snack list

DAY 4

Start the morning with half a lemon squeezed into warm water or cleansing herb tea. Follow with a brisk walk, bike ride, yoga or swimming

BREAKFAST: Coconut Banana Power Smoothie

100 grams of natural yoghurt or organic coconut milk, 1 tablespoon of cold pressed coconut oil, and 1 or 1/2 banana, 1 tablespoon of chia seeds. Blend the ingredients in a high speed blender.

LUNCH: 1 bowl of vegetable stew with a cup of quinoa or amaranth.

DINNER: Lentil and vegetable Stew.

ANY TIME SNACKS: Choose from the snack list

DAY 5

Start the morning with half a lemon squeezed into warm water or cleansing herb tea. Follow with a brisk walk, bike ride, yoga or swimming

BREAKFAST: Fresh vegetable juice with 1 table spoon of chia seeds blended in.

LUNCH: Steamed vegetables of choice with fresh herbs, drizzled with olive oil and crushed pumpkin seeds. Combine this with 1/2 cup organic brown rice and a handful of almonds

DINNER: Salad of fresh rocket leaves with thinly sliced strips of red capsicum, slices of fresh mushrooms and onions. Sprinkle with sunflower seeds. Toss with virgin olive oil, lemon and fresh herbs.

ANY TIME SNACKS: Choose from the snack list

DAY 6

Start the morning with half a lemon squeezed into warm water or cleansing herb tea.

Follow with a brisk walk, bike ride, yoga or swimming

BREAKFAST: Make a fruit compote of dried prunes, apricots, peaches and apples pre-soaked in filtered water and sprinkled with flaked almonds and 2 tablespoon of ground flaxseeds. Have it with some plain yogurt.

LUNCH: Lentil and vegetable soup with 1/2 cup of brown rice and amaranth.

DINNER: Raw Papaya and Carrot Salad

ANY TIME SNACKS: Choose from the snack list.

DAY 7

Start the morning with half a lemon squeezed into warm water or cleansing herb tea.

Follow with a brisk walk, bike ride, yoga or swimming

BREAKFAST: Coconut banana power smoothie

LUNCH: Lentil and vegetable soup with tossed greens, dressed with olive oil and a splash of lemon juice. Accompany with a handful of raw almonds and raisins.

DINNER: Grilled mushrooms with green salad, sweet potato mash and 1/2 cup of brown rice

ANY TIME SNACKS: Choose from the snack list

LIVER RESCUE DIET RECIPES

In this part are nourishing liver rescue diet recipes to help cleanse your liver and improve overall health.

Arugula, Potato, and Asparagus Salad

Preparation time

1 hour

Ingredients:

- 4 to 5 potatoes (about 3 cups roughly chopped)
- 1 cup chopped brussels sprouts
- 1 cup chopped asparagus
- 1/2 cup thinly sliced sweet onion
- 1/4 cup loosely packed fresh parsley, roughly chopped
- 1/4 cup roughly chopped fresh basil leaves
- 1 teaspoon dried thyme
- 2 tablespoons lemon juice
- 1 tablespoon pure maple syrup
- 4 cups arugula

• 2 cups chopped butter leaf, romaine, and/or green leaf lettuce

Instructions

1. To prepare the potatoes, add 3 inches of water to a medium-sized pot, bring it to a boil, and add a steaming basket.

2. Place the potatoes in the basket, cover, and steam for 15 to 20 minutes, until the potatoes are very tender.

3. To prepare the brussels sprouts, steam for 10 minutes, until tender.

4. To prepare the asparagus, steam for 5 minutes, until tender.

5. To streamline the above process, feel free to steam the potatoes, brussels sprouts, and asparagus together in one large basket. So that nothing gets overcooked, start by steaming the potatoes, then 5 to 10 minutes later, add the brussels sprouts. After another 5 minutes, add the asparagus.

6. Steam for an additional 5 minutes, or until all contents of the steamer basket are tender.

7. Remove the potatoes, brussels sprouts, and asparagus and place them in a large bowl.

8. Let them cool for 10 minutes, and then add the onion, parsley, basil, dried thyme, lemon juice, maple syrup, arugula, and lettuce.

9. Toss until evenly mixed.

10. Serve immediately.

Cauliflower Potato Mash

Preparation time

30 minutes

Ingredients:

- 4 to 5 medium-sized potatoes, peeled and roughly chopped*
- 1 small head of cauliflower, cut into large florets
- 2 teaspoons garlic powder
- 2 teaspoons onion powder

- 1 tablespoon chopped chives, parsley, or green onions, to serve
- 1/2 teaspoon paprika, to serve

Instructions

1. Add 3 inches of water to a medium-sized pot, bring it to a boil, and add a steaming basket.
2. Place the potatoes and cauliflower florets in the basket, cover, and steam for 15 to 20 minutes, until both are very tender.
3. Remove the potatoes and cauliflower and place them in a large bowl or pot.
4. Add the garlic powder and onion powder.
5. Mash until smooth using an immersion blender or potato masher.

6. Serve topped with chives, parsley, or green onions, and paprika.

Banana Salad

Preparation time

5 minutes

Ingredients:

- 1/2 cup thinly sliced onion (optional)
- 2 tablespoons to 1/4 cup Atlantic dulse strips, quickly soaked in water, then chopped
- 4 to 6 bananas, chopped

- 1 cup chopped cucumber (optional)
- 2 to 3 sticks celery, chopped (optional)
- 4 to 6 cups leafy greens (such as butter lettuce, romaine, and/or red leaf lettuce)

FOR THE DRESSING

- 2 teaspoons raw honey
- 1/2 cup orange juice

Instructions

1. Place the onion (if using), Atlantic dulse, bananas, cucumber (if using), celery (if using), and leafy greens in a medium-sized bowl.
2. Toss until evenly combined.

3. Whisk together the raw honey and orange juice in a small bowl.

4. Add to the salad and toss again.

5. Serve immediately.

Everything Bagels

Preparation time

40 minutes

Ingredients:

- 3 tbsp ground flax + 1/2 cup water
- 1/2 cup melted coconut oil

- 3 tbsp maple syrup
- 2 cups cassava flour
- 1/2 cup arrowroot starch
- 1 cup coconut flour
- 1/2 cup brown rice flour
- 2 1/2 tsp baking powder
- 1/3 cup + 1-2 tbsp water

Everything seasoning:

- 2 tbsp onion granules or flakes
- 2 tbsp garlic granules or flakes
- 2 tbsp black sesame seeds
- 2 1/2 tbsp white sesame seeds

- 1 tbsp poppy seeds
- 1 tsp flaked or regular sea salt (optional)

Instructions

1. Bring a large pot of water to boil.
2. Preheat oven to 430F/220C and line a baking sheet with parchment paper.
3. In a small bowl, whisk together the ground flaxseeds and water.
4. Let stand for 5 minutes.
5. Pour in the coconut oil and maple syrup and whisk until uniform.

6. Set aside. In a large bowl, add the cassava flour, arrowroot, coconut flour, brown rice flour and bak-ing powder.

7. Whisk until uniform and lump-free.

8. Pour in the wet ingredients and stir, adding water one tablespoon at a time, until the dough starts coming together.

9. Knead with your hands until you get a uniform, soft dough.

10. Shape the dough into balls, flatten slightly and make a hole in the middle using a chop-stick on your finger. The dough is quite crumbly, so smaller bagels will be easier to shape.

11. Gently submerge a bagel in boiling water and cook for 30 seconds on both sides.

12. Transfer to baking sheet and sprinkle Everything Seasoning on top.

13. Repeat with rest of dough.

14. Bake for 18-20 minutes, until lightly browned on top.

15. Transfer to wire rack and cool. These bagels taste best when still slightly warm. Best stored in an airtight container at room temperature.

Sweet Potato Tortilla Soup

Preparation time

45 minutes

Ingredients:

- 1 cup diced red or yellow onion, extra to serve
- 4 garlic cloves, minced
- 2 1/2 cups chopped fresh tomatoes
- 2 cups Healing Broth (recipe on page 368) or water
- 2 tablespoons tomato paste
- 1/4 to 1/2 teaspoon chipotle powder
- 1 teaspoon ground cumin

- 1 teaspoon ground coriander
- 1 teaspoon paprika
- 1 teaspoon pure maple syrup
- 1 cup diced sweet potato
- 1 1/2 tablespoons lime juice
- Fresh cilantro, to serve

Instructions

1. Place a large ceramic nonstick pot on medium-high heat and add the 1 cup of onion and the garlic.

2. Cook for 3 to 5 minutes, until the onion is translucent, adding a spoonful of water if needed.

3. Add the chopped tomatoes, Healing Broth or water, tomato paste, chipotle powder, ground cumin, ground coriander, paprika, and maple syrup.

4. Place the lid on and simmer for 20 minutes.

5. Add in the sweet potato and lime juice and cook for a further 10 to 15 minutes, until the sweet potato is very tender.

6. Divide between bowls and top with the extra onion and fresh cilantro.

7. Serve immediately.

Red Cabbage Tacos

Preparation time

15 minutes

Ingredients:

FOR THE TACOS

- 1 small head of red cabbage, broken into leaves
- 1 to 2 medium-sized tomatoes, diced
- 1/4 cup diced red onion
- 1/2 avocado, thinly sliced (optional)
- 1 red bell pepper, thinly sliced
- 1/4 cup loosely packed fresh cilantro, to serve

MANGO GINGER SAUCE

- 1 cup diced mango
- 2 tablespoons lime juice
- 1/2-inch piece of fresh ginger
- 1/4 to 1/2 teaspoon cayenne or red pepper flakes
- 2 medjool dates
- 3 tablespoons water

Instructions

1. Arrange cabbage leaves on plates or a platter and top with diced tomatoes, red onion, avocado

(if using), red bell pepper, and cilantro. Set aside.

2. Make the sauce by combining the mango, lime juice, ginger, cayenne or red pepper flakes, dates, and water in a blender.

3. Blend until smooth.

4. Spoon sauce onto the Red Cabbage Tacos.

5. Serve immediately.

Strawberry Banana Salad

Preparation time

15 minutes

Ingredients:

FOR THE SALAD

- 4 cups chopped strawberries
- 4 to 6 bananas, roughly chopped (about 4 to 6 cups)
- 4 cups leafy greens (such as spinach and/or butter leaf lettuce)
- 1/4 cup finely chopped basil or sage (optional)

ORANGE HONEY DRESSING (OPTION 1)

- 1/2 cup orange juice
- 2 teaspoons raw honey

STRAWBERRY BANANA DRESSING (OPTION 2)

- 1/3 cup chopped strawberries
- 1/3 cup chopped banana
- 1 to 3 tablespoons water
- 1 teaspoon lemon juice (optional)
- 2 basil leaves (optional)

Instructions

1. Place the strawberries, bananas, leafy greens, and basil or sage (if using) in a medium-sized bowl.

2. Gently toss until evenly combined.

3. If you're using the first dressing option, whisk together the orange juice and raw honey in a small bowl.

4. Add to the salad and gently toss again.

5. If you're using the second dressing option, combine the strawberries, banana, 1 tablespoon of water, lemon juice (if using), and basil (if using) in a blender and blend until very smooth. If you like a thinner consistency, add another 1 to 2 tablespoons of water.

6. Add to the salad and gently toss again.

7. Serve immediately.

Banana Nori Wraps

Preparation time

15 minutes

Ingredients:

- 4 nori sheets
- 2 cups alfalfa sprouts, divided
- 4 green onions
- 4 bananas (or 4 steamed potatoes, roughly chopped— see Tips)
- Atlantic dulse flakes, to taste

- 1/2 cup fresh cilantro (optional)

Instructions

1. Place a nori sheet shiny side down on a chopping board with a long edge close to you.
2. Arrange 1/2 cup sprouts, 1 green onion, 1 banana (or 1 chopped potato), dulse flakes, and cilantro (if using) on one end of the sheet.
3. Brush water across the other end of the sheet, and then roll it up tightly.
4. Cut in half and repeat with the remaining ingredients.
5. Serve immediately.

Sweet & Sour Stir Fry

Preparation time

20 minutes

Ingredients:

- 1/2 cup chopped green onions
- 1 cup sliced carrots
- 2 cups broccoli florets
- 2 cups chopped asparagus
- 1 cup thinly sliced bell peppers (red, orange, and/or yellow)

FOR THE SAUCE

- 1 cup unsweetened or fresh pineapple juice
- 2 tablespoons lime juice
- 1 teaspoon grated ginger
- 1 teaspoon grated garlic
- 1/4 to 1/2 teaspoon cayenne or red pepper flakes
- 2 tablespoons pure maple syrup
- 2 tablespoons tomato paste
- 1 tablespoon arrowroot powder

Instructions

1. In a medium-sized bowl, whisk together the pineapple juice, lime juice, grated ginger and

garlic, cayenne or red pepper flakes, maple syrup, tomato paste, and arrowroot powder. Set aside.

2. Add the green onions and carrots to a large non-stick ceramic pan.

3. Cook for 3 to 5 minutes, adding a bit of water if needed to prevent sticking, until the carrots are almost tender.

4. Add in the broccoli florets, asparagus, and bell peppers and cook for a further 5 minutes.

5. When all the vegetables are tender, pour in the sauce and bring it to a boil, stirring frequently, until thickened.

6. Remove from the heat and serve immediately.

Buffalo Cauliflower

Preparation time

45 minutes

Ingredients:

- 1 medium-sized head of cauliflower, cut into bite-sized florets
- 1 1/3 cup cassava flour
- 1 1/2 cup water, more if needed
- 6-8 celery sticks, to serve

Ranch:

- 1 cup raw, peeled and diced zucchini
- 2 tbsp raw cashews
- 1 tbsp lemon juice
- 1/2 tsp garlic powder
- 1 tsp onion powder
- 1/2 tbsp finely chopped dill
- 1/2 tbsp finely chopped parsley

Hot Sauce:

- 2-3 tbsp roughly chopped fresh red hot peppers
- 2 garlic cloves
- 2 1/2 tbsp lemon juice

- 1 tsp paprika
- 2 tbsp raw honey
- 3/4 cup water
- 1 tbsp arrowroot starch
- 1/4 cup tomato paste
- Celery stalks

Instructions

1. Preheat oven to 425F. Line a large baking sheet with parchment paper.

2. In a large bowl, whisk together the cassava flour and water. The batter should be thick enough to coat the cauliflower. If it's too thick, add a few tablespoons of water.

3. Add the cauliflower to the bowl and toss until well coated.

4. Using a fork, transfer the battered cauliflower to the baking sheet, shaking off the excess batter.

5. Leave at least 1 inch between each piece.

6. Place in the oven for 20-25 minutes, until crisp.

7. Flip the cauliflower pieces over halfway through.

8. To make the ranch sauce, combine the zucchini, cashews, lemon juice, garlic powder and onion powder in a blender and blend until smooth.

9. Stir in the dill and parsley and set aside.

10. To make the hot sauce, combine the fresh hot peppers, garlic, tomato paste, lemon juice, paprika, raw honey, water, and arrowroot starch in a blender.

11. Blend until smooth.

12. Pour the mixture into a large saucepan over medium-high heat and bring to a simmer. If the sauce is very thick add a bit more water.

13. Add the baked cauliflower and toss to coat.

14. Remove from heat and place on a serving plate or platter together with the celery stalks.

15. Serve immediately with prepared ranch sauce.

Liver Detox Smoothie

Preparation time

10 minutes

Ingredients

- 1 ripe banana, peeled*
- 1/2 green apple, cored and chopped
- 1 medium-sized carrot, peeled and chopped
- 1 handful baby spinach
- 1 (1/4-inch) nub turmeric root, peeled
- 1 Tbsp fresh parsley, chopped
- 3 walnut halves

- 2 Tbsp Hemp Protein Powder
- 1/2 lemon, juiced
- 1 pinch cinnamon, optional
- 3/4 cup unsweetened almond milk, see note**

Instructions

1. Add all ingredients for the smoothie to a blender and blend until completely smooth.
2. Taste smoothie for flavor and add more cinnamon and/or some honey to taste.

Liver Cleanse Soup

Preparation time

1 hour 15 minutes

Ingredients

- 3 cups filtered/purified water
- 1 cup organic vegetable broth
- 2 organic beets (peeled + diced)
- 2 organic carrots (sliced)
- 2 cups organic broccoli (chopped)
- 10 cloves organic garlic (freshly crushed)
- 1 organic onion (diced)

- 1/2 organic lemon (freshly squeezed)
- 2 organic bay leaves
- 1/2 teaspoon Himalayan pink salt
- 1/2 teaspoon organic ground turmeric
- 1/2 teaspoon organic dried oregano
- 1/2 teaspoon organic ground black pepper

Instructions

Prepare the veggies:

1. Slice/Dice/Cut the beets, carrots, broccoli, and onions to the size of your preference.

Prepare the soup:

1. Add all the ingredients for the soup to a medium-size pot and bring to a boil.

2. Lower the heat and simmer on low heat for approximately 1 hour, or until the veggies are soft.

3. Add extra water or veggie broth if needed and adjust seasonings to your preference.

Chickpea Quiche

Preparation time

1 hour 15 minutes

Ingredients

Chickpea Mix

- 3 cups of chickpea flour
- 2 cups of water
- 4 tbsp of fresh lemon juice
- 2 tbsp of poultry seasoning
- 2 teaspoons of salt
- 8 peeled garlic cloves

Filling

- 1 diced red onion
- 1 bag of frozen veggies I used a mix of broccoli, cauliflower and carrots

Instructions

1. Preheat the oven to 400ºF.

2. Defrost the vegetables according to the package instructions. Put all the ingredients of the chickpea mixture in the blender and blend until a smooth batter forms.

3. In a bowl mix the vegetables and onions with the chickpea mixture and pour in a baking dish.

4. Bake until the top is browned and when you insert a toothpick it comes out mostly clean, this will take between 40 to 60 minutes depending on the oven.

5. Allow cooling before serving and enjoy!

Celery Juice Recipe + Protocol

Preparation time

10 minutes

Ingredients

1 - 2 bunches organic celery

Instructions

Prep the celery:

1. Cut off the base of the celery and remove any leaves.

2. Wash / Rinse the celery with baking soda + purified / filtered water.

Juice the celery (with a juicer):

1. Place the celery stalk into the shoot of your juicer and juice according to the manufacturer's instructions.

2. Strain the juice until ALL pulp is removed.

3. Consume immediately or store in an air-tight glass container in the refrigerator overnight, but no longer than that.

Blend the celery (with a Vitamix):

1. Place the celery stalks in a Vitamix and blend until it becomes a liquid.

2. Using a nut milk bag, strain ALL the pump from the juice.

3. Consume immediately or store in an air-tight glass container in the refrigerator overnight, but no longer than that.

Sweet Potato and Carrot Soup

Preparation time

30 minutes

Ingredients

- 1/2 cup cooked lentils
- 1 sweet potato, peeled and cut in cubes

- 3 carrots, peeled and roughly chopped
- 1 parsnip, peeled and roughly chopped
- 1 onion, peeled and cut in quarters
- 3 garlic cloves, crushed
- 1 teaspoon turmeric powder
- 1 teaspoon cumin powder
- 1/4 teaspoon sea salt
- 2 cups low sodium vegetable broth, warm
- 1 teaspoon grated ginger
- 1 pinch chili powder
- 1 teaspoon coconut oil
- fresh parsley, flaxseed, toasted mixed nuts, coconut milk - to garnish

Instructions

1. Heat the oven at 165°C/329°F.

2. Line a baking sheet with baking paper, add the sweet potato, carrots, parsnip, onion, garlic, turmeric, cumin, chili, coconut oil, salt and toss to combine.

3. Roast for 20 minutes, then transfer into the blender.

4. Add the warm broth, grated ginger and cooked lentil and process to obtain a smooth cream

5. Serve warm, garnished with mixed nuts and seeds, parsley and coconut milk.

Delicious Detox Salad

Preparation time

35 minutes

Ingredients

For salad

- 1/2 medium sized head of red cabbage, shredded
- 3 carrots, coarsely grated
- 2 tbsp roughly chopped, fresh parsley
- 2 Gala apples, quartered, cored and sliced
- Handful of radishes or 2 celery sticks, sliced

- 3 tbsp toasted pine nuts
- 1 tbsp pumpkin seeds
- 2 tbsp sunflower seeds
- 2 tbsp flax seed

For dressing

- 2 tsp grated ginger root
- 1 tsp honey
- 2 tbsp fresh squeezed lemon juice
- 4 tbsp light olive oil

Instructions

1. For faster preparation of the salad ingredients use a food processor fitted with the shredding plate or use a mandolin.

2. Prepare all of the salad ingredients and mix them in a large bowl.

3. In a small bowl, whisk together all of the dressing ingredients until thickened.

4. Pour the dressing over the salad and toss to evenly coat.

5-Ingredient Liver Detox Juice

Preparation time

13 minutes

INGREDIENTS

- 1 beet, scrubbed
- One handful of greens, washed (dandelion greens are very good for the liver if you are ok with the bitter taste)
- 1 apple
- 1 cucumber, peeled
- 1 lemon, peeled
- 1 scoop Further Food Collagen Peptides
- Optional 1 scoop Superfood Turmeric

INSTRUCTIONS

1. Juice all ingredients, stir and enjoy!

DETOX VEGETABLE BROTH WITH TURMERIC AND GINGER

Preparation time

1 hour 30 minutes

Ingredients

- 1 gallon filtered water

- 1 large onion, roughly chopped
- 1 leek, roughly chopped (including tops)
- 4 cloves garlic, sliced in half
- 3 parsnips, roughly chopped
- 1 bunch parsley
- 1/2 head green cabbage, roughly chopped
- 1 3-inch piece of ginger, roughly chopped
- 3 celery stalks, roughly chopped
- 1 tablespoon ground turmeric
- Sea salt to taste

Instructions

1. Thoroughly wash and clean all of the vegetables. You do not need to peel any of the vegetables and aromatics for this broth, but it is up to you.

2. Peeling them (ginger, garlic, parsnips, onion) will give the broth a cleaner taste and appearance, but it is not necessary.

3. Combine all of the vegetables and the water into a large stock pot.

4. Bring to a simmer, cover with lid, and gently simmer for 90 minutes.

5. Strain the liquid through a fine mesh strainer and discard the vegetables.

6. Store in mason jars or airtight containers in the refrigerator for 1 week, or freeze.

7. Enjoy warm or use as a soup base or while making quinoa or rice.

Buckwheat Breakfast Muffins

Preparation time

25 minutes

Ingredients

- 1 cup buckwheat groats, soaked
- ½ cup unsweetened coconut flakes
- ¼ cup walnuts, chopped
- ¼ cup pumpkin seeds
- 2 Tbsp. chia seeds

- ¼ cup flaxseed meal
- 1 tsp. cinnamon
- ¼ tsp. salt
- 2 eggs
- 1 ½ cups almond milk
- ¼ cup almond butter
- 3 packets or 1 ½ tsp. powdered stevia
- 1 Tbsp. alcohol free vanilla
- Coconut milk, cinnamon, coconut flakes, walnuts and pumpkin seeds for garnish

Instructions

1. In a medium bowl, soak buckwheat groats with a pinch of salt overnight or about 6 to 7 hours.

2. Drain and rinse groats thoroughly with fresh water, drain again.

3. Preheat oven to 375 degrees F (190 degrees C).

4. Brush a 12 cup muffin tin generously with oil, such as coconut oil, set aside.

5. In a large bowl, add buckwheat groats, coconut flakes, walnuts, pumpkin seeds, chia seeds, flaxseed meal, cinnamon and salt, stir to combine.

6. In a small bowl, add eggs, almond milk, almond butter, stevia and alcohol free vanilla, whisk until frothy.

7. Pour liquid ingredients into bowl with dry ingredients, stir to combine.

8. Scoop about ⅓ cup muffin mixture into each cup of the prepared muffin tin.

9. Bake muffins for about 15 to 20 minutes or until muffins have browned around the edges and are firm to the touch.

10. Cool muffins in tin for about 10 minutes.

11. Serve warm with coconut milk, a dusting of cinnamon and a garnish of coconut flakes, walnuts and pumpkin seeds.

MINI CHICKPEA QUICHES

Preparation time

55 minutes

Ingredients

- 4 cups frozen broccoli florets – thawed and chopped, or use fresh
- 4 cups grape tomatoes
- 1 large red onion – diced
- 8 cloves of garlic – cut off ends by the stem, but leave the skin on
- 2 cups water

- 3 cups chickpea flour (garbanzo bean flour)
- 1 lemon – juiced
- 2 tsp poultry seasoning
- 2 tsp Himalayan cooking salt

Instructions

1. Preheat oven 400ºF
2. Spread broccoli, tomatoes, onion, and garlic cloves on 2 parchment-lined baking sheets and roast 15-20 minutes or until tender
3. Peel the roasted garlic – careful, it will be hot – and add it to a blender with the water, chickpea flour, lemon juice, poultry seasoning, and salt and blend until a smooth batter forms

4. Pour batter into a large mixing bowl and stir in the remaining roasted vegetables

5. Use a ladle to spoon batter into a standard 12-cup silicone muffin pan (or use a metal muffin pan lined with parchment baking cups)

6. Bake for 30-35 minutes or until the tops are brown and a toothpick inserted in the middle comes out clean

7. Allow to cool before serving

Easy Oven Roasted Potatoes

Preparation time

50 minutes

INGREDIENTS

- 4 large potatoes peeled & cubed
- 1 tbsp coconut oil melted
- 1 tsp sea salt
- 1 tsp onion powder
- 1 tsp garlic powder
- 1 tsp paprika

INSTRUCTIONS

1. Preheat oven to 400F.

2. Melt coconut oil and set aside.

3. Line baking sheet with parchment paper.

4. Place cubed potatoes in a large bowl.

5. Add sea salt, onion powder, garlic powder and paprika.

6. Stir to coat potato cubes.

7. Add melted coconut oil.

8. Stir to coat.

9. Spread potato cubes out in single layer on baking sheet.

10. Bake for 40 minutes, until potatoes are browned and cooked through.

Pink pickled rhubarb with ginger

Preparation time

20 minutes

Ingredients

- white wine vinegar 200ml
- caster sugar 100g
- ginger a few peeled slices
- yellow mustard seeds 2 tsp
- sea salt 1 tsp
- pink rhubarb 400g, cut into diagonal pieces
- bay leaves 2 small

Instructions

1. Put the vinegar, sugar, ginger, mustard seeds and sea salt in a pan with 200ml water.

2. Heat until the sugar dissolves, then simmer for 2 minutes. Cool to room temperature.

3. Sterilise a large jar by washing it in hot soapy water, rinsing and putting it in an oven heated to 160C/fan 140C/gas 3 for 10 minutes.

4. Put the rhubarb and bay leaves in the jar, then pour over the liquid (including the ginger and seeds).

5. Put in the fridge and leave for a couple of days before eating.

Liver Detox Smoothie

Preparation time

5 minutes

Ingredients

- 1 inch of fresh turmeric
- ½ cup raw shredded beets
- 1 packed cup raw spinach leaves
- ½ a fresh apple, or ½ cup unsweetened apple sauce
- 1 cup frozen cherries
- 2 tablespoons chia seeds

• 1 cup unsweetened almond milk, milk of choice, or coconut water

• Juice of ½ or 1 full lemon, depending on your preference

Instructions

1. Roughly chop turmeric and apple, and shred beets with a cheese grater.

2. Add all ingredients to a blender and blend on high until completely smooth.

3. Best tasting when enjoyed immediately, but stays pretty well in the fridge over night if you want to prep ahead.

Liver Cleansing Carrot Cake

Preparation time

55 minutes

INGREDIENTS

- 1 cup plain flour
- 3/4 teaspoon baking soda
- 1 teaspoon baking powder
- 1/2 teaspoon cinnamon
- 1/2 teaspoon nutmeg
- 1/2 teaspoon salt
- 3/4 cup raw sugar

- 2 eggs
- 1/3 cup cold pressed oil
- 2 teaspoons cold pressed oil
- 1 cup grated carrot
- 440g crushed pineapple, drained
- 1/4 cup chopped walnuts

Instructions

1. Preheat oven to 350f.
2. Mix together all ingredients but carrot pineapple and walnuts.
3. Fold in carrot, pineapple and walnuts.
4. Pour into greased and lined tin. Bake for 35-40 minute.

Oatmeal Raisin Cookies

Preparation time

35 minutes

Ingredients

- 2 tablespoons flax seeds (ground golden)
- 6 tablespoons water
- 1 1/2 cups gluten-free rolled oats
- 1 cup gluten free oat flour
- 2 tablespoons coconut sugar
- 1/2 teaspoon baking powder

- 1/2 baking soda
- 1 teaspoon ground cinnamon
- 1/4 teaspoon sea salt
- 1/4 cup coconut oil
- 1/3 cup maple syrup
- 1 teaspoon alcohol (free vanilla extract)
- 3/4 cup raisins (organic)

Instructions

1. Preheat oven to 350F.
2. Line a baking sheet with parchment paper.
3. Mix together the ground flax seeds and water to make the flax egg.

4. Leave to soak for 15 minutes

5. In a medium-sized bowl, combine the oats, oat flour, coconut sugar, baking powder, baking soda, cinnamon and sea salt. Mix until uniform.

6. In another bowl, whisk together the avocado oil, maple syrup, vanilla and flax egg.

7. Add to the dry ingredients and stir until you get a uniform batter.

8. Stir in the raisins.

9. Using a large cookie scoop, scoop the mixture and drop onto the parchment paper.

10. Flatten into round disks using a fork.

11. Place in the oven and bake for 10-12 minutes, until slightly browned.

12. Remove from the oven and cool.

Apple Crumble With A Difference

Preparation time

35 minutes

Ingredients

- 4 large apples, peeled, cored and diced
- 2 cups cooked quinoa
- 1 cup flour
- 1/2 chopped cashews, walnuts, or pecans
- 1/3 cup ground almonds
- 2 teaspoons cinnamon

Instructions

1. Preheat oven to 350 degrees.

2. Lightly oil (e.g. extra virgin olive oil or coconut oil) 13″x9″ baking dish or 6 ramekins.

3. Place apples into prepare dish(es).

4. Mix remaining ingredients in medium bowl and crumble over the top of the apples.

5. Bake for 30 minutes or until apples are tender and crumble is lightly browned.

Tomato Detox Soup

Preparation time

1 hour 15 minutes

Ingredients

- 1 pint grape tomatoes
- 1 TBS grapeseed or olive oil
- 1 TBS chopped ginger
- 1/2 cup chopped Vidalia onion
- 3 cloves garlic minced 2 TBS or garlic paste
- 2 14.5 ounce cans fire-roasted diced tomatoes
- 1- quart vegetable stock

- Handful of fresh Basil
- Kosher salt & black pepper
- Optional: for heat, add a few pinches of cayenne pepper
- Optional: 1/2 TBS sugar
- Optional: fresh basil leaves
- Garnish: Pepitas

Instructions

1. Heat your oven to 300 degrees.
2. Place tomatoes in a small baking dish or in some aluminum foil (with the top open) and roast them for 35 minutes.

3. Turn off the oven and allow them to sit in the oven for an additional 15 minutes.If you are running out, they can sit there until cool. You can do this a day ahead if you like)

4. When ready to make the soup.

5. Heat oil in a medium pot, saute onions and ginger for a few minutes, add in garlic and roasted tomatoes and saute for a couple more minutes, you can press down on the tomatoes with the back of a spoon or a potato masher to "pop" them if you like.

6. Add canned tomatoes and vegetable stock, season and bring to a simmer.

7. Simmer for 10 minutes, add in Basil and season some more until you get the taste you desire.

8. Decide if you want to puree your soup or leave it chunky (I like it mostly pureed). Using an immersion blender or traditional blender/Vitamix. Puree soup.

9. Enjoy hot, room temperature or cold.

10. Garnish with a handful of pepitas (pumpkin seeds), chives or scallions and Basil and enjoy!

The Perfect Lunch Salad

Preparation time

10 minutes

INGREDIENTS

- 3 handfuls mixed greens or spinach

- 3 radishes, sliced
- ½ cucumber, sliced
- ½ avocado, cubed
- 1-2 green onions, sliced thin (to taste)
- 1 tbsp sunflower or pumpkin seeds (to taste) *see tip at the bottom
- ½ lemon, juiced
- 1 handful sprouts (optional)
- sea salt, herbamare, and/or pepper to taste

Instructions

- Mix it all up, drizzle the lemon juice on top, and pack it in a container for lunch or serve immediately.

Mango Fruit Salad with Coconut Flakes, a great summer dessert

Preparation time

10 minutes

INGREDIENTS

- 1200 grams mangoes (approximately 4 ripe mangoes – 42.33oz)
- 250 grams blueberries (approximately 2 small punnets – 8.82oz)
- 1 cup coconut flakes toasted
- 1 medium lime, juice

INSTRUCTIONS

1. Peel the mango, cut into dice and remove the pit.

2. Rinse your blueberries in a colander under cold running water and shake dry.

3. Place all the salad ingredients in a large mixing bowl and mix until well combined.

4. Serve chilled with lime sorbet to counteract the sweetness of the mangoes.

WHITE BEAN STEW

Preparation time

45 minutes

Ingredients

- 6 cups white beans of choice - boiled I used small white beans
- 3 tomatoes - chopped
- 1 medium onion - chopped
- 5 garlic cloves - minced
- ¼ stem of leeks - chopped
- 1 teaspoon ground white pepper

- 3 small stock cubes (Maggi) about 3.5 g cubes optional
- ½ cup oil I used corn oil
- 1 carrot - chopped
- Salt

Instructions

1. Pour oil in a pot and heat on medium heat. Add in onions and saute until translucent.
2. Add in tomatoes and fry stirring all the time until it starts sticking to the pot.
3. Add in garlic and stir until fragrant.
4. Add in the leeks, white pepper and carrots then stir.

5. Add a cup of water (or stock if you happen to have some), stock cubes and salt to taste.

6. Stir well and let simmer for 2 minutes,

7. Add beans and mix to combine with the stew.

8. Let it simmer for about 5 minutes.

9. Add more water if you like it watery but if you like it thick, leave as it is.

10. Taste to ensure that the seasoning is perfect.

11. Serve with boiled rice or with any side of choice.

Vegan Blueberry Banana Bread

Preparation time

50 minutes

INGREDIENTS

- 3 ripe bananas
- 1/4 cup pure maple syrup
- 1/4 cup coconut sugar
- 1 tsp vanilla extract
- 1/2 cup unsweetened almond coconut milk
- 1 1/2 cups gluten free oat flour
- 1/2 cup arrowroot starch

- 1/2 tsp sea salt
- 1 tsp aluminum free baking powder
- 1/2 tsp baking soda
- 1/2 cup frozen wild blueberries
- chopped walnuts, for topping optional

INSTRUCTIONS

1. Preheat oven to 350 degrees. Line a 9x5 loaf pan with parchment paper.

2. Mash bananas in a bowl with fork or potato masher.

3. Add maple syrup, coconut sugar, vanilla extract and almond coconut milk. Mix well.

4. In a separate bowl, combine oat flour, arrowroot starch, sea salt, baking powder, and baking soda.

5. Add wet ingredients and stir gently, until ingredients form a batter. Add frozen blueberries and fold in very gently, stirring just until mixed in.

6. Pour batter into loaf pan.

7. Top with walnuts, if desired, and bake in oven for 40 minutes.

8. Then turn off oven and leave blueberry banana bread in oven for another 10 minutes.

9. Remove from oven and cool completely, on a rack, before slicing. Serves 4.

Detox Spinach Soup

Preparation time

20 minutes

Ingredients

- 100 gr spinach
- 1 big carrot cut into small pieces
- ½ pepper cut into dices
- 1 onion cut into dices
- 2 garlic minced
- ¼ cup leek chopped
- 2 cups vegetable broth

- 2 cups water
- 1 tbsp olive oil
- Salt
- Black pepper

Instructions

1. Heat a big soup pot over medium heat.
2. Toss the olive oil, the onion, and the garlic and cook until the onion is semi-transparent.
3. Toss the carrot, the pepper, the spinach and the leek.
4. Cook until the spinach loses a lot of water and reduces in size.
5. Pour the vegetable broth and the water.

6. Simmer for 15 minutes until the carrot is soft.

7. Blend the soup and add salt and black pepper to taste.